Pregnancy Workout Guide

Workout Routine For Every Trimester From First to Third

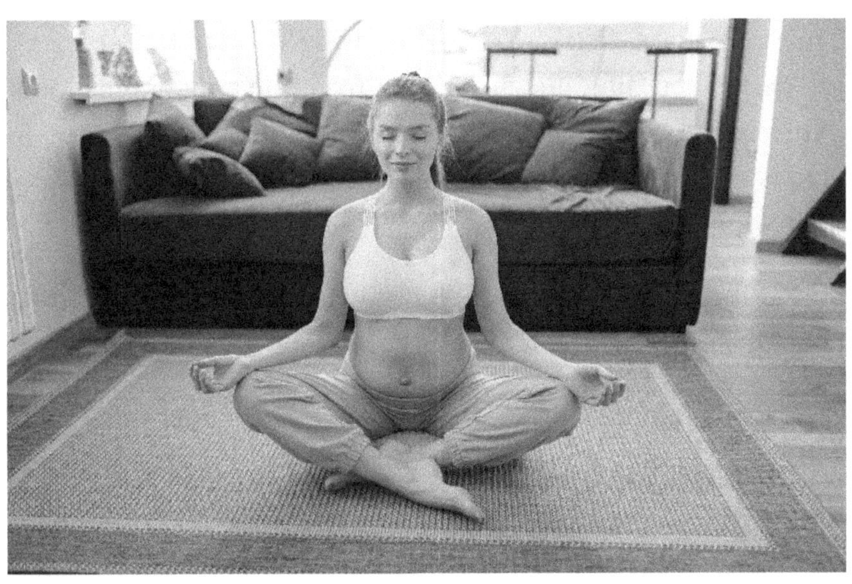

Thomas P. Tinney

Contents

Chapter One

1.0 Introduction to Pregnancy Fitness

Maria was happy to find out she was pregnant, but she knew she needed to keep healthy for herself and her developing baby. She decided to hunt for a pregnant fitness plan to assist her in keeping healthy and active throughout her Pregnancy.

She came onto a book named "Pregnancy Workout Handbook" and quickly purchased it. As soon as it came, she quickly went through the pages and was delighted with the content. The book addressed everything from the advantages of exercising during Pregnancy to safe and effective routines for each trimester.

Maria was resolved to put the book's suggestions into action. Throughout her first trimester, she performed the suggested cardio and strength training workouts, which helped her remain motivated and reduced her morning sickness. She also learned how to adapt her exercises as her Pregnancy developed.

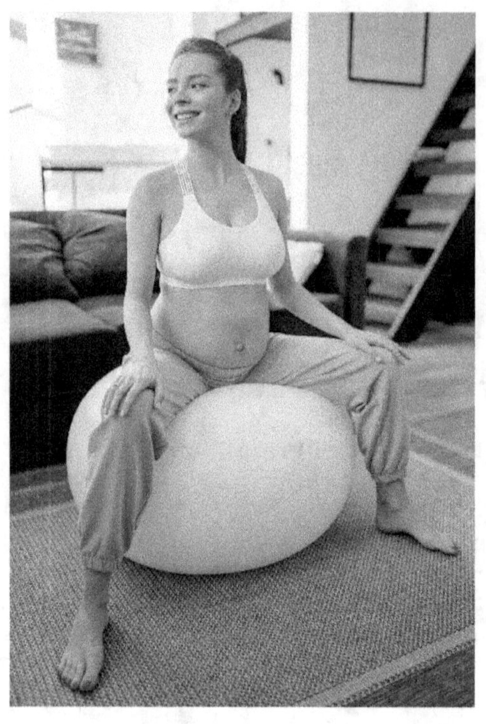

When she approached her second trimester, Maria introduced prenatal yoga and Pilates into her practice, which helped her relax and prepare for labor and Delivery. She continued exercising frequently and felt confident in her body's ability to manage the changes.

Maria was thankful for the book's workout adaptations and Breathing exercises instructions in her third trimester. She also learned how to conduct pelvic floor exercises to prepare for Delivery.

Eventually, the day came for Maria to deliver her baby. She recalled the book's advice on practicing core exercises throughout labor and found it helpful during Delivery. Due to the "Pregnancy Workout Guide," Maria could keep healthy and active throughout her Pregnancy and felt secure throughout her birth.

When she held her lovely baby in her arms, Maria felt thankful for the assistance the book had given her throughout her pregnancy journey.

Introduction to Prenatal Fitness is crucial for every pregnant mother trying to be healthy and active throughout Pregnancy. Exercising during Pregnancy offers various advantages, including increased mood, lower risk of gestational diabetes and hypertension, and excellent sleep quality. But, exercising during Pregnancy also demands some care and attention to safety.

Expectant moms should contact their healthcare practitioners before commencing any fitness program, especially if they have any previous medical issues. Some workouts and activities should be avoided, such as contact sports or routines that involve laying on your back for a lengthy time. The intensity and frequency of exercise should also be modified to match the demands of each lady.

The exercise suggested during Pregnancy often includes low-impact aerobic, strength training, and flexibility activities, such as prenatal yoga and Pilates. These exercises may be customized to each trimester and can help prepare women for Delivery.

Prenatal Fitness is a fantastic approach to keeping healthy throughout Pregnancy and preparing for Delivery. By following the recommendations and guidance of healthcare practitioners and implementing safe and practical activities into their routines, pregnant moms may enjoy the numerous advantages of exercise during Pregnancy while protecting the health and safety of both themselves and their developing kids.

1.1 Benefits of exercising during Pregnancy

Exercising during Pregnancy has several advantages, both for the mother and the baby. These are some of the primary benefits:

- **Decreased risk of gestational diabetes:** Exercising during Pregnancy may help manage blood sugar levels and lower the risk of gestational diabetes, which is a kind of diabetes that arises during Pregnancy.

- **Reduced risk of hypertension:** Exercise has been demonstrated to lessen the chance of having high blood pressure during pregnancy, which may be risky for both the mother and the baby.

- **Increased mood:** Exercise has been linked to enhanced mood and decreased anxiety and sadness, which may be particularly useful during pregnancy when hormonal changes can induce mood swings.

- **Improved sleep quality:** Frequent exercise may enhance sleep quality and minimize the chance of developing sleep problems during Pregnancy.
- **Decreased back discomfort:** Many pregnant women have back pain, which may be improved by strengthening the core and back muscles via exercise.

- **Increased stamina and endurance:** Exercise may assist in boosting endurance and stamina, which can be advantageous during labor and Delivery.

- **Improved weight management:** Regular exercise during Pregnancy may help regulate weight increase and avoid excessive weight gain, which can lead to health concerns.

- **Decreased risk of premature labor:** Studies have indicated that regular exercise throughout Pregnancy may lessen the risk of preterm labor and Delivery.

- **Increased fetal health:** Regular exercise during Pregnancy has been related to enhanced fetal health, including a decreased risk of fetal macrosomia (a condition in which the infant is more significant than typical) and improved cardiovascular health.

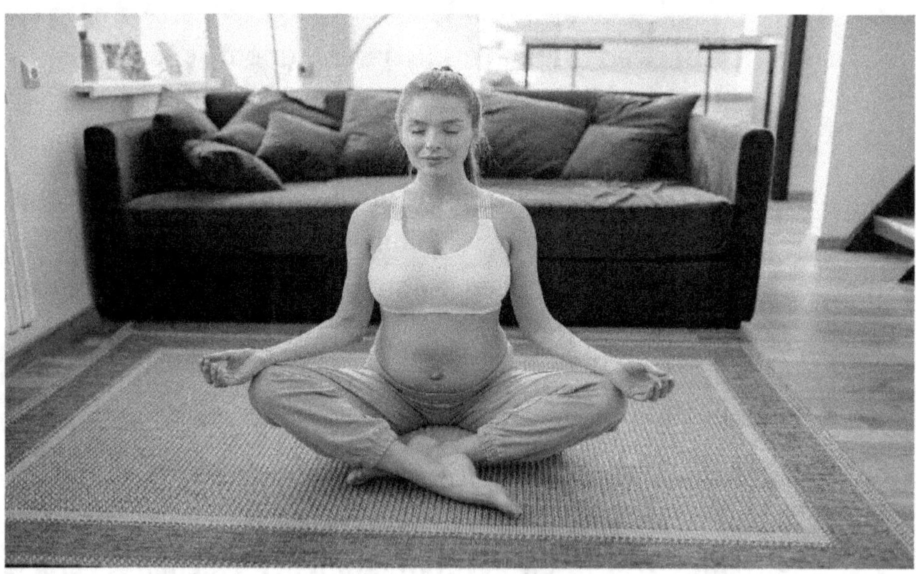

Overall, the advantages of exercise during Pregnancy are enormous and far-reaching. Women who frequently exercise throughout Pregnancy may enhance their health and wellness and their developing kids. Nonetheless, contacting a healthcare physician before commencing any fitness program during Pregnancy is vital to ensure safety and efficacy.

1.1.1 Decreased risk of gestational diabetes:

Gestational diabetes is a kind of diabetes that develops during Pregnancy. It may lead to health concerns for both the mother and the baby, including an increased chance of developing type 2 diabetes later in life. Nevertheless, frequent activity throughout Pregnancy may help minimize the chance of developing gestational diabetes.

Exercise helps manage blood sugar levels and may enhance insulin sensitivity, which can help avoid gestational diabetes. In addition, exercise may help limit weight gain during Pregnancy, a risk factor for developing gestational diabetes.

One research indicated that women who participated in at least 30 minutes of moderate-intensity exercise most days of the week had a 50% decreased chance of acquiring gestational diabetes compared to those who were less active.

It is crucial to emphasize that women with a history of gestational diabetes, obesity, or other risk factors for gestational diabetes should check with their healthcare professionals before commencing any fitness program during Pregnancy. In certain circumstances, further monitoring or measures may be essential.

Overall, exercise is an excellent approach to minimizing the risk of gestational diabetes and enhancing general health throughout Pregnancy. Women who are pregnant or expecting to get pregnant should examine the benefits and dangers of exercise during Pregnancy with their healthcare professionals to identify the best strategy for their unique requirements.

1.1.2 Reduced risk of hypertension

Hypertension, or high blood pressure, is a common illness that may be harmful during Pregnancy. It may lead to problems such as preeclampsia, a dangerous illness that can damage both the mother and the baby. Nonetheless, frequent activity throughout Pregnancy may help minimize the chance of developing hypertension.

Exercise helps increase blood circulation and may minimize the risk of high blood pressure. In addition, exercise may help control weight gain during Pregnancy, a risk factor for developing hypertension.

One study found that women who engaged in moderate-intensity exercise for at least 150 minutes per week had a 24% lower risk of developing hypertension during pregnancy than those who were less active.

It is important to note that women with a history of hypertension or other medical conditions should consult with their healthcare provider before beginning any exercise program during Pregnancy. In certain circumstances, further monitoring or measures may be essential.

Overall, exercise effectively reduces the risk of hypertension during Pregnancy and improves overall health. Women who are pregnant or expecting to get pregnant should examine the benefits and dangers of exercise during Pregnancy with their healthcare professionals to identify the best strategy for their unique requirements.

1.1.3 Improved mood:

Pregnancy can be a time of great joy and excitement, but it can also be a time of stress and anxiety. Hormonal changes, physical discomfort, and the anticipation of childbirth can contribute to mood swings and negative emotions. However, regular exercise during Pregnancy can help improve mood and reduce anxiety and depression.

Exercise has been shown to stimulate the release of endorphins, which are natural feel-good chemicals in the brain. This can lead to improved mood and reduced stress and anxiety. In addition, exercise can provide a sense of accomplishment and control, which can help counteract feelings of helplessness or overwhelm.

One study found that women who exercised regularly during Pregnancy reported less anxiety and depression than those who were less active. In addition, women who continued to exercise after giving birth reported better mood and overall well-being.

It is important to note that women with a history of depression or other mental health conditions should consult with their healthcare provider before beginning any exercise program during Pregnancy. In some cases, additional support or treatment may be necessary.

Overall, exercise is an effective way to improve mood and reduce stress and anxiety during Pregnancy. Women who are pregnant or expecting to get pregnant should examine the benefits and dangers of exercise during Pregnancy with their healthcare professionals to identify the best strategy for their unique requirements.

1.1.4 Enhanced sleep quality:

Getting enough sleep during Pregnancy can be challenging, as physical discomfort, hormonal changes, and anxiety can interfere with sleep quality. However, regular exercise during Pregnancy can help improve sleep quality and reduce the likelihood of sleep disturbances.

Exercise has been shown to improve sleep by promoting relaxation and reducing stress and anxiety. In addition, exercise can help regulate the circadian rhythm, the internal clock that controls sleep and wake cycles.

One study found that women who exercised regularly during Pregnancy reported better sleep quality and fewer sleep disruptions than those who were less active. In addition, women who continued to exercise after giving birth reported improved sleep quality and fewer insomnia symptoms.

It is vital to remember that women should avoid strenuous activity close to bedtime since this might interfere with sleep. Listening to your body and adapting your workout program to prevent overexertion or injury is also crucial.

Exercise is an excellent way to promote sleep quality during Pregnancy and improve overall health. Women who are pregnant or expecting to get pregnant should examine the benefits and dangers of exercise during Pregnancy with their healthcare professionals to identify the best strategy for their unique requirements.

1.1.5 Increased stamina and endurance

Being physically active throughout Pregnancy will assist in building stamina and endurance, which can be advantageous during labor and Delivery. Frequent exercise may help prepare the body for the physical demands of childbirth and may lessen the need for medical interventions during Delivery.

Exercise has been demonstrated to enhance cardiovascular endurance, muscular strength, and physical Fitness. This may help decrease weariness and enhance energy levels, which can be particularly essential during the latter stages of Pregnancy.

One research indicated that women who participated in regular exercise during Pregnancy had better endurance levels and could exercise longer than those who were less active. In addition, women who continued to exercise after birth reported greater energy levels and improved physical functioning.

It is crucial to highlight that women should avoid high-impact or intense activity during Pregnancy, particularly during the latter stages when the body is under more significant pressure. Listening to your body and adapting your workout program to prevent overexertion or injury is also crucial.

Overall, exercise is a great technique to boost stamina and endurance throughout Pregnancy and prepare the body for Delivery. Women who are pregnant or expecting to get pregnant should examine the benefits and dangers of exercise during Pregnancy with their healthcare professionals to identify the best strategy for their unique requirements.

1.1.6 Increased fetal health

Frequent exercise throughout Pregnancy has been found to have a favorable influence on fetal health. Exercise may promote average fetal growth and development by improving healthy blood flow and oxygen delivery to the baby.

Research has indicated that women who exercise regularly throughout Pregnancy have a decreased chance of having a baby with low birth weight. Low birth weight is connected with an increased risk of developmental issues, therefore increasing fetal growth and development is an essential objective for pregnant moms.

In addition, exercise during Pregnancy has been demonstrated to enhance fetal heart rate variability, which is a sign of fetal welfare. This implies that regular exercise might assist in maintaining a healthy pregnancy and contribute to excellent fetal outcomes.

It is crucial to highlight that women should contact their healthcare physician before commencing any workout regimen during Pregnancy. In certain circumstances, exercise may need to be reduced or avoided owing to particular medical issues or consequences.

Overall, exercise during Pregnancy is a safe and effective strategy to maintain fetal health and promote healthy growth and development. Women who are pregnant or expecting to get pregnant should examine the benefits and dangers of exercise during Pregnancy with their healthcare professionals to identify the best strategy for their unique requirements.

1.2 Safety concerns for exercising while pregnant

Although exercising during Pregnancy is typically safe and healthy, there are specific safety issues that should be taken into mind.

Speaking with a healthcare physician before commencing any fitness regimen during Pregnancy is crucial. Women with specific medical issues or consequences may need to avoid or alter some forms of exercise.

Secondly, listening to your body and preventing overexertion or pushing yourself too hard is crucial. Workouts should be pleasant and not cause any pain or discomfort.

Thirdly, some forms of activity should be avoided during Pregnancy, such as contact sports or activities with a high risk of falls or injury. They include soccer, basketball, skiing, and horseback riding.

Fourthly, women should avoid exercising in hot or humid surroundings, which might raise the risk of dehydration and overheating. It is crucial to be well-hydrated throughout the exercise and take pauses if required.

Finally, women should be cautious of altering the center of gravity and balance throughout Pregnancy. Actions involving many leaping, bouncing, or rapid movements should be avoided.

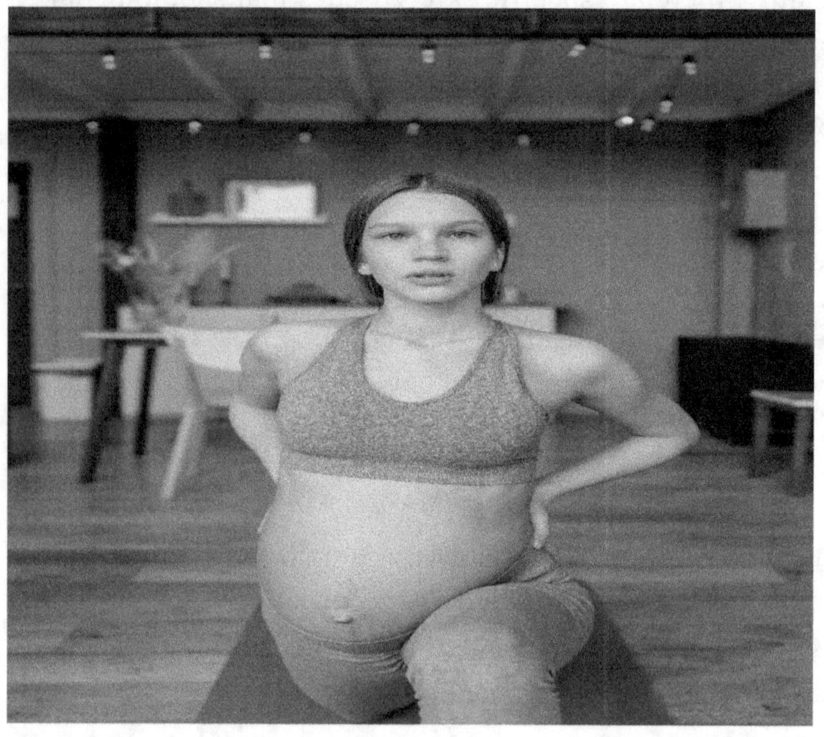

In summary, exercising during Pregnancy may be safe and valuable, but it is vital to consider certain safety factors. Women should talk with their healthcare practitioner, listen to their bodies, avoid certain forms of activity, be well-hydrated, and be careful of their shifting center of gravity and balance.

1.3 Varieties of exercise advised during Pregnancy

Numerous forms of exercise are typically safe and encouraged during Pregnancy. They include:

1. **Low-impact aerobic exercise:** This includes activities such as walking, swimming, and cycling. These exercises are gentle on the joints and may assist in enhancing cardiovascular health and endurance.

2. **Strength training:** This includes activities such as weightlifting, bodyweight exercises, and resistance band workouts. Strength training may enhance muscular strength and tone, which can be advantageous during labor and Delivery.

3. **Yoga and Pilates:** These forms of exercise assist in increasing flexibility, balance, and relaxation. They may also help decrease stress and boost mood.

4. **Pelvic floor exercises:** Commonly known as Kegels, pelvic floor exercises may help strengthen the muscles that support the bladder, uterus, and rectum. This may be particularly advantageous during and after Pregnancy.

5. **Prenatal fitness courses:** These sessions are mainly developed for pregnant women and may involve aerobic activity, strength training, and stretching.

It is crucial to highlight that women should contact their healthcare physician before commencing any workout regimen during Pregnancy. In certain circumstances, exercise may need to be reduced or avoided owing to particular medical issues or consequences.

A mix of low-impact aerobic activity, weight training, yoga or Pilates, and pelvic floor movements into a regular fitness regimen may be safe and valuable throughout Pregnancy. Women who are pregnant or expecting to get pregnant should review the forms of exercise that are safe and suggested for their unique requirements with their healthcare professionals.

1.3.1 Low-impact aerobic activity

Low-impact aerobic exercise is a sort of exercise that is mild on the joints and may be helpful during Pregnancy. It incorporates constant exercise that elevates the heart rate and enhances cardiovascular health without exerting too much stress on the body.

Some forms of low-impact aerobic activity that are safe and encouraged during Pregnancy include:

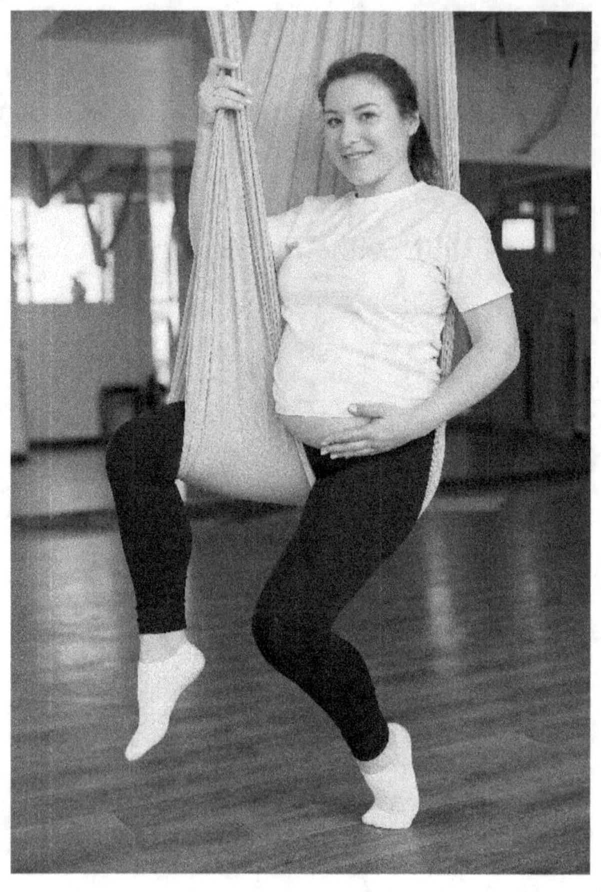

- **Walking:** This is one of the most accessible types of exercise and can be done anywhere. Walking may improve cardiovascular health, raise energy levels, and decrease stress.

- **Swimming or water aerobics:** These kinds of exercise benefit pregnant women since they support the body's weight and limit the danger of damage. Swimming or water aerobics may improve cardiovascular health, muscular tone, and flexibility.

- **Cycling:** Cycling is another low-impact aerobic activity that might be useful during Pregnancy. It may assist in enhancing cardiovascular health and endurance while minimizing the chance of joint harm.

- **Dancing:** Dancing is a pleasant and low-impact approach to increasing the heart rate and promoting cardiovascular health. Prenatal dancing lessons are offered in many places and are particularly intended for pregnant mothers.

Listening to your body and preventing overexertion while participating in a low-impact aerobic activity during Pregnancy is vital. Women who are pregnant or expecting to become pregnant should talk with their healthcare professional before starting any fitness program and discuss which forms of exercise are safe and advised for their unique requirements.

1.3.2 Strength training

Strength training is a form of exercise that includes resistance to grow and tone muscles. Exercise may be safe and advantageous during Pregnancy, as it can assist in enhancing muscular strength and endurance, which can be helpful during labor and Delivery.

Some examples of strength training workouts that are safe and encouraged during Pregnancy include:

1. **Bodyweight exercises:** These include exercises such as squats, lunges, push-ups, and planks. They utilize the weight of the body to strengthen and tone muscles.

2. **Resistance band workouts:** Resistance bands are elastic bands that produce resistance when stretched. They may be used for a range of workouts, incorporating bicep curls, shoulder presses, and leg extensions.

3. **Weightlifting**: Weightlifting with modest weights may assist in developing muscular strength and tone. Women who are pregnant should avoid lifting big weights that might strain the back or abdomen.

Adopting good form and technique while participating in strength exercises during Pregnancy is crucial. Women who are pregnant or expecting to become pregnant should talk with their healthcare professional before starting any fitness program and discuss which forms of exercise are safe and advised for their unique requirements. In certain situations, adaptations may need to be made to particular workouts to meet the body's changing demands during Pregnancy.

1.3.3 Yoga and Pilates

Yoga and Pilates are popular kinds of exercise that may be useful for pregnant women. Both kinds of exercise emphasize Breathing, relaxation, and moderate movements that may assist in increasing strength, flexibility, and general Fitness.

Yoga is an exercise that originated in ancient India and included holding positions while concentrating on Breathing and meditation. Some examples of yoga positions that are safe and recommended for pregnant women include:

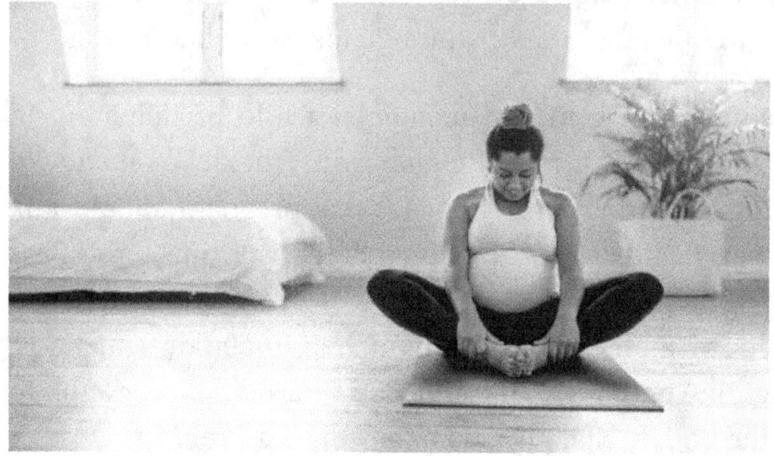

- **Cat-cow stance:** This pose includes alternating between arching and rounding the back while on all fours. It may enhance flexibility in the spine and reduce lower back discomfort.

- **Tree posture:** This position includes standing on one leg with the other foot placed on the opposite thigh. It may assist in enhancing balance and strength in the legs.

- **Child's posture:** This position requires kneeling on the ground with the arms held out in front of the body. It may help reduce stress and tension in the back and shoulders.

- **Pilates** is a style of exercise that focuses on strengthening the core muscles, improving posture, and developing flexibility. Some examples of Pilates exercises that are safe and suggested for pregnant women include:

- **Pelvic tilts:** This exercise includes reclining on the back with the legs bent and the feet flat on the ground. It includes shifting the pelvis forward and backward to strengthen the abdominal muscles.

- **Leg circles:** This exercise includes laying on the side with the legs straight and elevating one leg in the air while creating tiny circles with the foot. It may assist in increasing strength and flexibility in the legs and hips.

- **Modified plank:** This exercise includes holding a plank posture on the hands and knees rather than on the hands and toes. It may assist in developing the core muscles without placing too much pressure on the body.

Women who are pregnant or expecting to become pregnant should talk with their healthcare professional before starting any fitness program and discuss which forms of exercise are safe and advised for their unique requirements. In certain circumstances, adaptations may need to be made to specific postures or exercises to meet the body's changing demands during Pregnancy.

1.3.4 Yoga and Pilates

Pelvic floor exercises, often known as Kegel exercises, are a kind of exercise that may be especially useful for pregnant women. These workouts target the muscles that support the pelvic organs, including the uterus, bladder, and colon.

The pelvic floor muscles may weaken during Pregnancy and Delivery, leading to complications such as incontinence and prolapse. Pelvic floor exercises may strengthen these muscles and lower the likelihood of these issues.

To practice pelvic floor exercises, follow these steps:

- **Name the pelvic floor muscles:** These are the muscles you employ to halt the flow of pee or avoid passing gas. You may also imagine squeezing the muscles you would use to hold in a tampon.
- **Tighten and raise the pelvic floor muscles:** Compress the pelvic floor muscles and pull them upward as though you are attempting to lift them into your body.
- Hold the contraction for 5-10 seconds: Hold the contraction for a few seconds, then release.
- **Repeat the exercise:** 10-15 times, three times each day.

Whether sitting, standing, or lying down, pelvic floor exercises may be done at any moment. It is vital to avoid holding your breath while executing the exercise and to relax the muscles between contractions.

Women who are pregnant or expecting to become pregnant should talk with their healthcare professional before starting any fitness program and discuss which forms of exercise are safe and advised for their unique requirements. Pelvic floor exercises are usually considered safe during Pregnancy. However, adaptations may need to be made in specific circumstances.

1.3.5 Prenatal fitness classes:

Prenatal fitness courses are sessions mainly intended for pregnant women to help them keep active and healthy throughout Pregnancy. These sessions are generally conducted by licensed fitness experts who are informed about pregnant women's unique demands and limits.

Prenatal fitness programs may provide a range of advantages for pregnant women, including:

- **Professional assistance:** Prenatal exercise courses are guided by experienced fitness experts who can instruct safe and practical activities during Pregnancy.

- **Social support:** Joining a prenatal fitness class may give a chance for pregnant women to connect with others who are going through a similar experience, which can be helpful for both physical and mental well-being.

- **Customized workouts:** Prenatal fitness programs are intended to meet the changing demands of pregnant women, including changes for various stages of Pregnancy and considerations for any medical issues.

- **Motivation:** Being part of a group may incentivize you to keep active and commit to a regular fitness regimen.

Prenatal fitness programs may take numerous forms, including yoga, Pilates, low-impact aerobics, and strength training. Several fitness clubs and studios offer pregnancy exercise programs, and online choices are accessible for individuals who want to work out at home.

Before starting any prenatal fitness program, it is crucial to contact a healthcare physician to confirm that it is safe for you and your baby. Also, it is crucial to listen to your body and make adaptations as required to ensure that you exercise safely and successfully.

Chapter Two

2.0 First Trimester Workouts

Vivien was ecstatic when she found out that she was pregnant. Being a fitness lover, she was determined to maintain her routines during Pregnancy. But, throughout her first trimester, she found it tough to acclimatize to the changes in her body.

She endured periods of nausea and lethargy that left her feeling depleted and uninspired. Despite this, she continued to push herself to maintain her workout program. She lowered the intensity and length of her workouts, concentrating on low-impact activities such as walking and swimming.

Vivien also added strength training routines that targeted the main muscular groups. She was careful to listen to her body and take breaks when required, remaining hydrated and eating a balanced meal to fuel her exercises.

One day, while completing a set of squats, Vivine felt a searing discomfort in her lower abdomen. She immediately stopped exercising and checked with her healthcare professional, who recommended she rest and avoid vigorous exercise for a few days.

Vivien was scared that she had hurt her baby. Still, her healthcare professional reassured her that it was typical to have some pain during Pregnancy and that listening to her body and making alterations as required was essential.

With time, Vivien learned to adapt to the bodily changes of her first trimester and continued to stay active throughout her Pregnancy. She discovered that exercise helped her manage stress and improve her general happiness, and she was delighted to bring her kid into a healthy and active lifestyle.

The first trimester of Pregnancy is a period of considerable changes in a woman's body. It may be tough to adapt to physical changes while maintaining activity and health. Yet, being active throughout the first trimester is vital for physical and mental well-being. Here are some concerns and guidelines for first-trimester workouts:

- **Talk with a healthcare professional:** Before starting any fitness program, it is crucial to contact a healthcare practitioner to confirm that it is safe for you and your baby. In certain circumstances, alterations may need to be made depending on medical history or present conditions.

- **Listen to your body:** Throughout the first trimester, many women suffer symptoms such as exhaustion, nausea, and breast soreness. It is vital to listen to your body and alter your routines appropriately. For example, if you are feeling exhausted, lower the intensity or length of your exercises.

- **Select low-impact workouts:** During the first trimester, avoiding high-impact exercises that might place additional pressure on the joints and ligaments is typically suggested. Instead, concentrate on low-impact workouts such as walking, swimming, and cycling.

- **Include strength training**: Strength exercise may assist in preserving muscle mass and increase overall strength and endurance. Throughout the first trimester, it is usually okay to continue with comfortable strength training activities that do not place additional pressure on the body. Concentrate on exercises that target the primary muscular groups, such as squats, lunges, and upper body workouts.

- **Perform pelvic floor exercises:** Pelvic floor exercises, commonly known as Kegels, may help strengthen the pelvic floor muscles and minimize the risk of incontinence and other issues. These workouts may be done throughout Pregnancy and are safe for most women.

- **Keep hydrated:** It is crucial to remain hydrated throughout Pregnancy, particularly during activity. Be sure to drink lots of water before, during, and after exercises.

- **Take breaks when required:** It is crucial to take breaks when needed and heed your body's cues. If you feel dizzy, lightheaded, or have any other troubling symptoms, stop exercising and rest.

Being active throughout the first trimester may enhance physical and mental well-being during Pregnancy. It is crucial to listen to your body and make adaptations to ensure that you exercise safely and successfully.

2.1 Activities to reduce morning sickness

Morning sickness, nausea, and vomiting are typical symptoms experienced by many pregnant women. Although there is no one-size-fits-all answer, several activities may help ease these symptoms and make Pregnancy more pleasant. These are some exercises that treat morning sickness:

1. **Deep Breathing:** Slow, deep Breathing may help relax your body and mind. Choose a peaceful spot, sit comfortably, and take deep breaths through your nose and out through your mouth.

2. **Yoga:** Several yoga positions may help relieve nausea and vomiting. Attempt moderate stretches such as the sitting forward bend, the child's posture, or the cat-cow stance.

3. **Walking**: A quick stroll will help get your blood circulating and lessen the sensations of nausea. Start with short walks and progressively expand your time and distance.

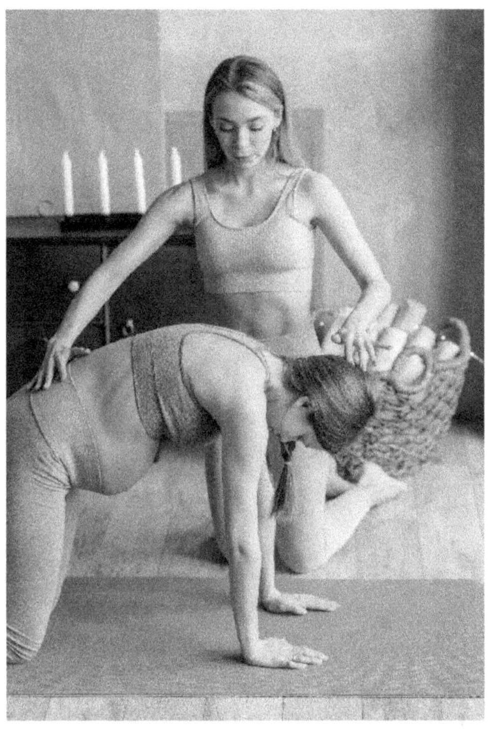

4. **Swimming:** Water is a relaxing environment that may help minimize nausea and vomiting. Swimming is a low-impact workout that may be done throughout Pregnancy.

5. **Pelvic tilts:** This exercise includes laying on your back and gently swaying your pelvis back and forth. It may help ease the strain on the lower back and minimize symptoms of nausea.

Always listen to your body and avoid workouts that cause discomfort or suffering. If morning sickness is severe or persistent, ask your healthcare professional for further help and direction.

2.2 Safe cardio exercises during Early Pregnancy

Cardiovascular activity is vital to a healthy pregnancy, but picking safe and low-impact workouts throughout early Pregnancy is crucial. These are some safe aerobic exercises for early Pregnancy:

- **Brisk walking:** Walking is an excellent low-impact cardio workout that may be done throughout Pregnancy. It's a terrific method to increase your heart rate and boost your cardiovascular health.
- **Swimming:** Swimming is a mild, low-impact workout on joints and muscles. It's a terrific way to keep active while lowering the chance of injury.

- **Stationary cycling**: Cycling on a stationary bike is a safe and effective technique to increase your heart rate throughout early Pregnancy. It's low-impact and can vary the resistance to meet your fitness level.
- **Low-impact aerobics:** Low-impact aerobics sessions are meant to be safe for pregnant women. These include motions that maintain at least one foot on the ground at all times, which decreases the danger of falls and injury.
- **Dancing:** Dancing is a fun and low-impact approach to increasing your heart rate during early Pregnancy. You might join a dancing class, especially for pregnant women, or dance to your favorite home music.

Always listen to your body and avoid workouts that cause discomfort or suffering. It's also crucial to remain hydrated and take breaks as required. If you have concerns about your fitness program during early Pregnancy, check with your healthcare practitioner for extra information.

2.2.1 Brisk walking:

Brisk walking is an effective low-impact exercise with various health advantages, particularly during Pregnancy. It's a simple but powerful technique to enhance cardiovascular health, develop muscular strength and endurance, and raise mood and energy levels.

During Pregnancy, brisk walking is a safe and recommended exercise that may help maintain a healthy weight, minimize the risk of gestational diabetes, and enhance general well-being. It's also a terrific approach to preparing your body for labor and Delivery.

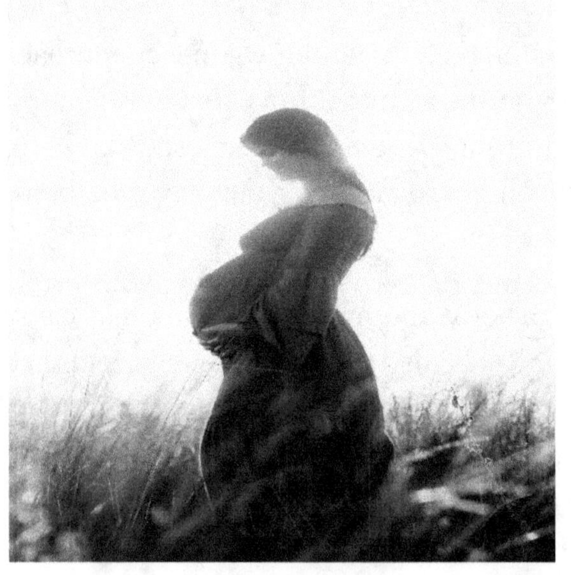

Aim for at least 30 minutes of moderate-intensity exercise most days of the week to get the most benefit of brisk walking. It's crucial to wear comfortable and supportive shoes and gear and to keep hydrated during your walk. If you're new to exercising, start softly and gradually increase your speed and length over time.

Brisk walking may be done anywhere, at any time, making it a handy and accessible form of exercise for pregnant women. Whether you like to stroll around your neighborhood, in a park, or on a treadmill at home or the gym, brisk walking is a low-impact and beneficial method to keep active throughout Pregnancy.

As with any activity during Pregnancy, it's vital to contact your healthcare professional to verify that brisk walking is healthy for you and your baby. Depending on your health state and pregnancy advancement, they may give specific advice and instructions.

2.2.2 Swimming

Swimming is a popular type of exercise for pregnant women since it delivers a full-body workout with minimum pressure on joints and muscles. It's a low-impact aerobic exercise that may enhance cardiovascular health, muscular strength and endurance, and general well-being during Pregnancy.

One of the primary advantages of swimming during Pregnancy is that it may help decrease pregnancy-related discomforts such as back pain, edema, and exhaustion. The buoyancy of the water may assist in supporting the weight of the developing baby, easing the strain on the joints and allowing for more range of movement. Swimming may also help regulate body temperature, which is vital during Pregnancy to prevent overheating.

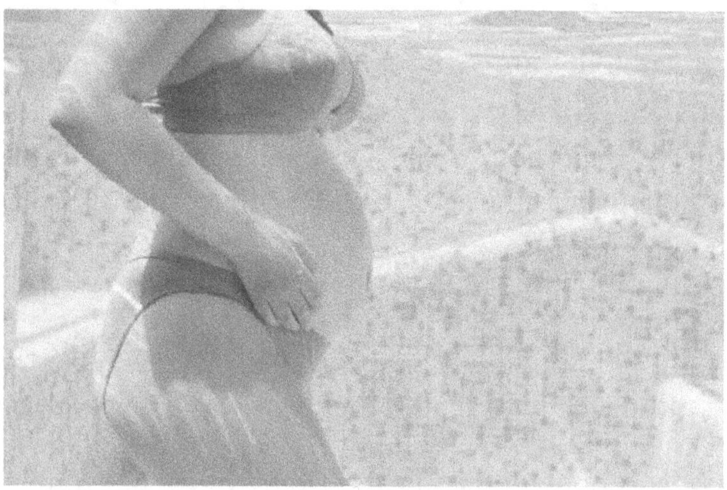

Swimming may be done during all stages of Pregnancy, but specific changes may be required as the belly becomes more considerable. For example, swimming on your side rather than your stomach may be more comfortable, or using a pool noodle or floating device for increased support.

To get the most out of swimming during Pregnancy, striving for at least 30 minutes of moderate-intensity activity most days of the week is suggested. It's crucial to wear comfortable and supportive swimwear and to keep hydrated during your swim. It's also a good idea to avoid swimming in open bodies of water containing hazardous germs or pollution.

Like any activity during Pregnancy, it's vital to contact your healthcare professional to verify that swimming is safe for you and your baby. Depending on your health state and pregnancy advancement, they may give specific advice and instructions.

2.2.3 Stationary cycling

Stationary cycling, often known as indoor cycling or spinning, is a popular kind of low-impact aerobic exercise that may be healthy for pregnant women. It delivers a rigorous exercise that may assist in improving cardiovascular health, leg strength, and endurance while being easy on the joints and muscles.

One of the primary advantages of stationary cycling during Pregnancy is that it's a low-impact exercise that may help ease discomforts such as back pain, edema, and exhaustion. It's also an excellent alternative for women who may not be able to engage in weight-bearing exercises owing to joint discomfort or other concerns.

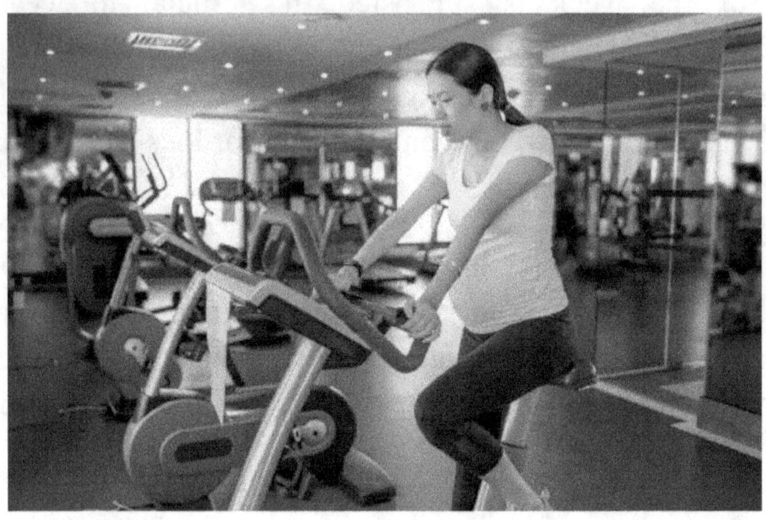

Stationary cycling may be done during all stages of Pregnancy, but changes may be required as the belly becomes more considerable. For example, riding a recumbent bike rather than an upright cycle or altering the seat and handlebars for greater comfort may be more pleasant.

To get the most out of stationary cycling during Pregnancy, striving for at least 30 minutes of moderate-intensity activity most days of the week is suggested. It's crucial to wear comfortable and supportive sports attire and to keep hydrated during your activity. It's also a good idea to avoid high-intensity intervals or standing climbs that may place too much pressure on the abdominal muscles.

As with any activity during Pregnancy, it's crucial to contact your healthcare professional to verify that stationary cycling is safe for you and your baby. Depending on your health state and pregnancy advancement, they may give specific advice and instructions.

2.2.4 Low-impact aerobics

Low-impact aerobics is a sort of cardio exercise that may be useful for pregnant women since it is mild on the joints and muscles. It incorporates motions that maintain one foot on the ground at all times, lessening the stress on the body.

Low-impact aerobics can improve cardiovascular health, build muscles, and enhance endurance. It may also help relieve discomforts such as back pain, edema, and exhaustion during Pregnancy.

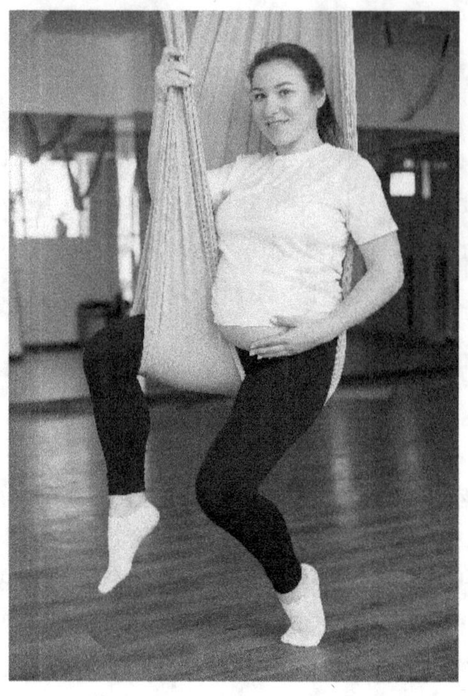

Low-impact aerobics include walking, cycling, swimming, Dancing, and prenatal aerobics sessions. These routines may be customized to suit each individual's fitness level and physical capabilities.

It's suggested that pregnant women try at least 30 minutes of moderate-intensity activity most days of the week. It's crucial to wear comfortable and supportive sports attire and to keep hydrated during your activity.

With low-impact aerobics, avoiding high-impact actions such as leaping or hopping is vital, which may place too much pressure on the abdominal muscles. It's also crucial to avoid workouts that involve laying on your back for a long time, particularly during the first trimester, since this might block the blood supply to the uterus.

As with any exercise during Pregnancy, you must contact your healthcare practitioner to verify that low-impact aerobics is safe for you and your baby. Depending on your unique health state and pregnancy advancement, they may give specific advice and instructions.

2.2.5 Dancing

Dancing is a fun and joyful kind of exercise that may be a terrific method for pregnant women to be active and healthy. Dancing may be a low-impact and moderate-intensity exercise that helps improve cardiovascular Fitness, build muscles, and increase balance and coordination.

Pregnant women may engage in various dancing disciplines, including ballet, hip-hop, jazz, ballroom, and Zumba. Prenatal dancing lessons are also offered in many places and are mainly intended to cater to pregnant women's unique demands and skills.

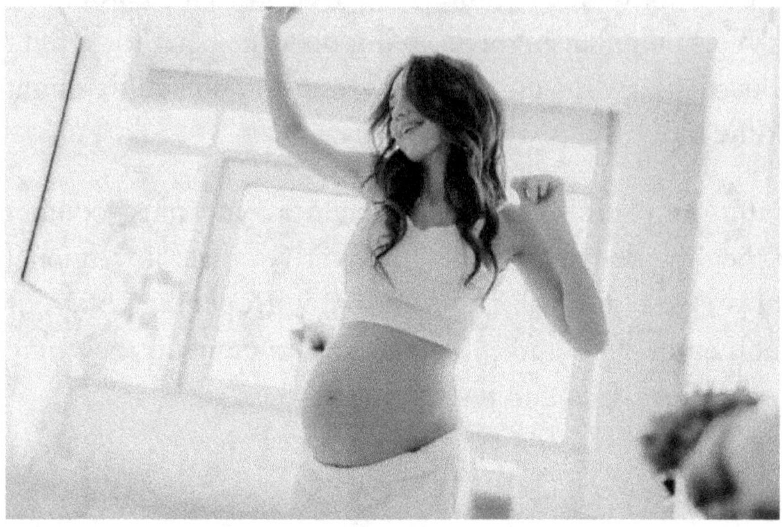

Dancing may be adapted to meet each individual's fitness level and physical capabilities. It's crucial to wear comfortable and supportive sports gear and proper shoes, such as dancing sneakers or low-heeled shoes.

While dancing during Pregnancy, it's crucial to avoid high-impact motions that might raise the risk of falls or injury. It's also vital to avoid workouts that entail considerable twisting, hopping or rapid changes in direction that might strain the abdominal muscles.

Pregnant women should always listen to their bodies and avoid pushing themselves too much. Whenever any discomfort or pain is encountered while Dancing, taking a break and relaxing is necessary.

Like any activity during Pregnancy, it's vital to contact your healthcare professional to verify that Dancing is healthy for you and your baby. Depending on your health state and pregnancy advancement, they may give specific advice and instructions.

2.3 Strength training exercises for the first trimester

Strength training routines might be good for pregnant women throughout the first trimester to help preserve muscle mass and develop strength. Yet, it's vital to approach strength training with prudence and take particular steps to safeguard the safety of both the mother and the baby.

Here are some safe and efficient strength training activities during the first trimester of Pregnancy:

- **Squats:** Squats are an excellent workout for strengthening the legs and glutes. Throughout the first trimester, avoiding squatting too deeply or carrying large weights is vital.

- **Lunges:** Lunges are another excellent workout for strengthening the legs and glutes. These may be changed by grabbing a firm surface for balance and support.

- **Sitting row:** Seated rows assist in strengthening the upper back and shoulders. It's vital to avoid stressing the abdominal muscles throughout this workout.

- **Chest press:** Chest presses help strengthen the chest and arms. Using lesser weights and avoiding laying flat on the back after the first trimester is recommended.

- **Bicep curls:** Bicep curls assist in strengthening the arms. Using lesser weights and avoiding stressing the abdominal muscles during this workout is vital.

While conducting strength training activities during the first trimester, utilizing modest weights and preventing overexertion is vital. It's also crucial to avoid holding your breath or straining the abdominal muscles. It's encouraged to undertake these exercises under the instruction of a professional prenatal fitness instructor or healthcare practitioner.

2.3.1 Squats

Squats are a favorite strength training activity that may be done safely throughout Pregnancy, especially in the first trimester. They efficiently target the lower body muscles, such as the glutes, quadriceps, and hamstrings.

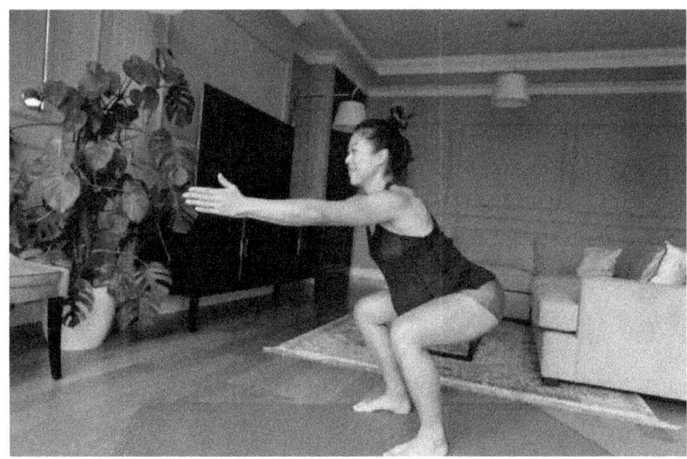

During the first trimester, squats may be done with bodyweight or extra resistance like dumbbells or resistance bands. Nonetheless, it is crucial to employ good form and technique to reduce lower back and pelvis tension.

To do a squat:

1. Stand with your feet hip-width apart and your toes pointed forward.
2. Engage your core and keep your back straight as you lower your body by bending your knees and hips as if sitting back onto a chair.
3. Keep your weight in your heels, and avoid letting your knees extend over your toes.
4. Wait for a bit before pushing through your heels to stand back up.

It is recommended to start with 1-2 sets of 10-12 repetitions and gradually increase as your body adapts to the exercise. As with any activity during Pregnancy, listening to your body and avoiding any motions or postures that create discomfort or suffering is crucial.

2.3.2. Lunges

Lunges are another excellent strength training exercise that may be done throughout the first trimester of Pregnancy.

They target the lower body muscles, including the quadriceps, hamstrings, and glutes.

Stand with your feet hip-width apart to perform a lunge and take a step forward with one foot. Maintain your chest raised and your shoulders back as you bend your knees and descend your body toward the ground. Your front knee should be precisely over your ankle while your rear knee hangs just above the ground. Press through your front heel to stand back up and repeat on the opposite side.

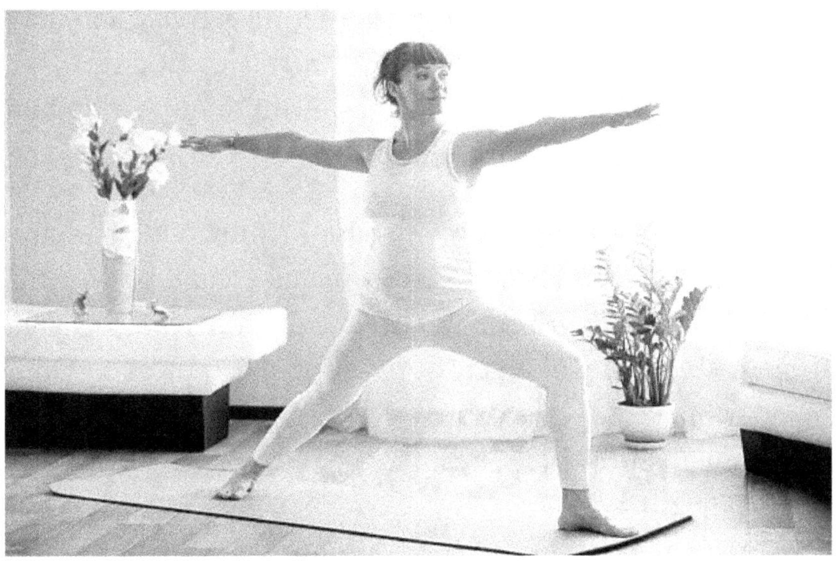

Maintaining appropriate form during lunges minimizes tension in the lower back or pelvis. Maintain your weight on your front heel and prevent your front knee from stretching past your toes. You may also adjust the workout by taking a shorter stride or holding onto a firm surface for support.

Similar to squats, it is advisable to start with 1-2 sets of 10-12 repetitions and progressively increase as your body adjusts to the activity. As usual, listen to your body and avoid any actions or postures that create discomfort or suffering.

2.3.3. Sitting row

The seated row is another strength training activity that may be done during the first trimester of Pregnancy. It targets the upper back and shoulders, helping to improve posture and lessen the risk of back discomfort.

Sit on a solid chair or bench with your feet flat on the ground to execute a seated row. Hold a resistance band or weights with an overhand grip and stretch your arms before you. Bring the band or weights towards your chest, pressing your shoulder blades together. Drop your arms back down to the beginning position and repeat.

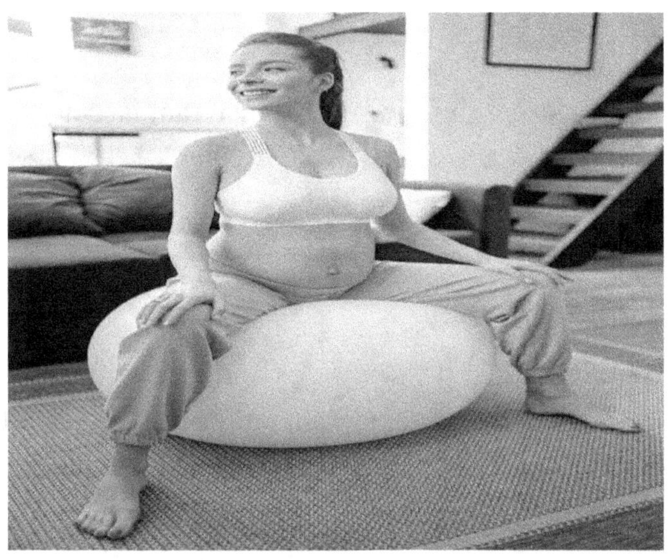

Maintaining proper posture throughout the sitting row is vital, as keeping your chest high and your shoulders relaxed. Avoid curving your back or hunching your shoulders forward since this might cause tension in the lower back.

Like any strength training exercise, starting with a lesser resistance and progressively increasing as your body adjusts to the activity is advisable. Try for 1-2 sets of 10-12 repetitions, pausing as required. While utilizing a resistance band, ensure it is adequately secured to a sturdy surface to prevent mishaps.

2.3.4 Chest press

The chest press is a strength training exercise that targets the chest, shoulders, and arms muscles. It involves pressing a weight away from the chest while lying on a bench, using a set of dumbbells or barbells.

During Pregnancy, chest press can be a safe and effective exercise to strengthen the chest muscles and improve upper body strength. However, choosing an appropriate weight that allows for proper form and avoids straining the muscles or joints is essential.

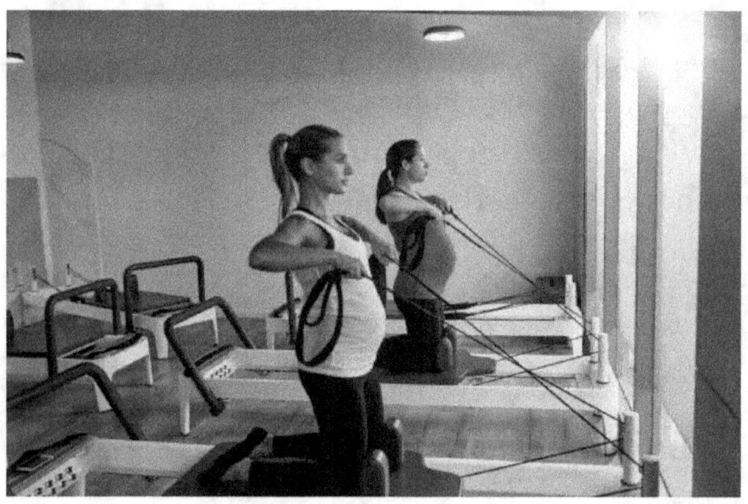

To perform a chest press during Pregnancy:

1. Lie on a bench or a stability ball with your feet flat.

2. Hold the dumbbells or barbells with your hands slightly wider than shoulder-width apart.
3. Gently lower the weights toward your chest, keeping your elbows tight to your torso.
4. Stop for a second, then push the weights back up to the starting position.

Breathing deeply during the activity and avoiding holding your breath are crucial. Stop immediately and talk with your healthcare physician if you suffer any discomfort or pain throughout the activity.

2.3.5 Bicep curls

Bicep curls are a typical strength training exercise that may be safely done during Pregnancy, particularly in the first trimester. This exercise mainly targets the biceps, the muscles positioned in the front of the upper arm.

You will need a set of dumbbells or resistance bands to execute bicep curls. Begin by standing with your feet shoulder-width apart and holding the dumbbells or resistance bands in each hand with your palms facing up. Hold your elbows close to your sides and steadily bring the weights towards your shoulders, bending at the elbow. Hold the posture for a time, then gently drop the weights back to your starting position.

It is crucial to pick a suitable weight to exercise in perfect form without straining. Start with a lesser weight and progressively raise as your strength increases.

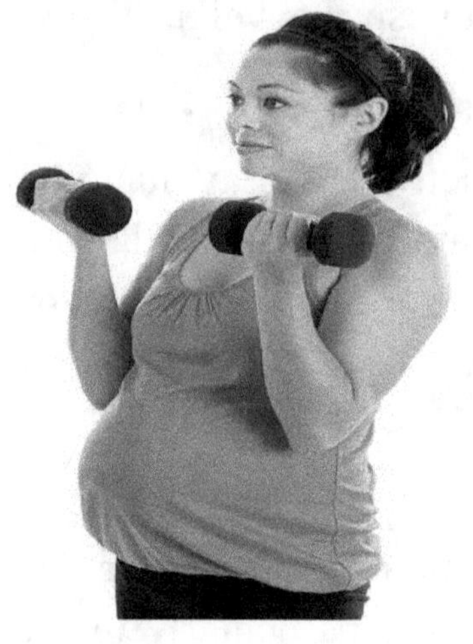

Like any activity during Pregnancy, listening to your body and not pushing yourself too hard is crucial. If you encounter discomfort or pain while practicing bicep curls or other workouts, stop immediately and talk with your healthcare physician.

Chapter Three

3.0 Second Trimester Workouts

3.1 Advantages of exercising during the second trimester

The second trimester is sometimes called the "honeymoon period" of Pregnancy. Around this period, many women notice a reduction in morning sickness and lethargy, giving it a perfect time to focus on exercise. There are various advantages to exercising during the second trimester, including:

1. **Better cardiovascular health:** As your baby develops, your heart needs to work harder to deliver blood to you and your growing baby. Frequent exercise throughout the second trimester may help strengthen your heart and enhance your overall cardiovascular health.

2. **Decreased risk of gestational diabetes:** Regular exercise during Pregnancy has been found to lessen the risk of gestational diabetes, a form of diabetes that develops during Pregnancy.

3. **Improved sleep:** Regular exercise may help improve sleep quality during Pregnancy, which is crucial for your and your baby's health.

4. **Improved muscle tone and strength:** Strength training activities, in particular, may help you maintain or even enhance muscle tone and strength throughout Pregnancy, aiding labor and Delivery and postpartum recovery.

5. **Better mood and decreased stress:** Exercise is a natural mood enhancer and may help reduce tension and anxiety during Pregnancy.

6. **Decreased risk of some pregnancy issues:** Regular exercise throughout Pregnancy has been found to lessen the risk of preeclampsia and gestational hypertension, two potentially significant pregnancy disorders.

7. **Preparing for labor and Delivery:** Some activities, like pelvic floor exercises and squats, may help prepare your body for labor and Delivery.

It's essential to remember that every Pregnancy is different, and it's always a good idea to talk with your healthcare professional before beginning or maintaining an exercise regimen during Pregnancy. But, for most women, exercising throughout the second trimester may be a safe and effective strategy to promote a healthy pregnancy.

3.2 Suggested cardio routines for the second trimester

During the second trimester of Pregnancy, aerobic activities may be an excellent approach to maintaining a healthy weight, decreasing stress, and enhancing cardiovascular health. Nonetheless, it's crucial to pick safe and suitable workouts for the pregnancy stage. These are some suggested aerobic routines during the second trimester:

1. **Elliptical machine:** This low-impact exercise is gentle on the joints and gives a full-body workout. It also enables you to regulate the intensity level.

2. **Stationary bike:** Like the elliptical machine, a stationary bike gives low-impact exercise and is customizable to your fitness level.

3. **Swimming:** Swimming is a terrific method to get full-body exercise without placing any stress on the joints. It's also an excellent alternative for discomfort or soreness during a workout.

4. **Brisk walking:** Walking is a simple and effective strategy to begin actively during Pregnancy. It's low-impact and may be done anywhere.

5. **Dancing:** If you like dancing, it may be a pleasant and low-impact approach to get your heart rate up. Make sure you pick low-impact types, such as ballroom or line dancing.

6. **Low-impact aerobics:** These courses are created exclusively for pregnant women and give a safe and effective method to begin exercising.

Remember to constantly listen to your body and alter your routines as required. Talking with your healthcare physician before beginning any new fitness program during Pregnancy is vital.

3.2.1 Elliptical machine

The elliptical machine is a popular exercise equipment commonly advised for pregnant women throughout their second trimester. This low-impact activity helps maintain cardiovascular Fitness and improve endurance without placing stress on the joints.

One of the perks of utilizing the elliptical machine is that it is simple to modify the difficulty and slope, enabling you to adapt your exercise to your fitness level and demands. Also, many machines feature grips you may grab onto for increased stability and support, which can be very useful as your belly swells.

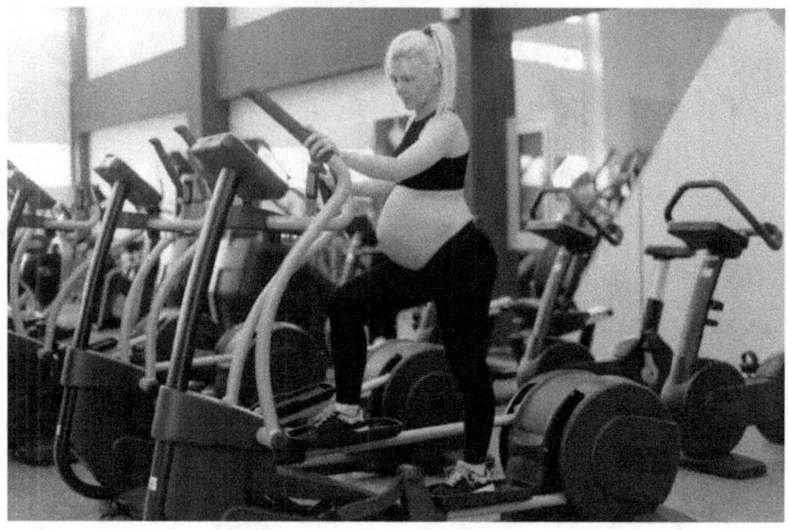

While utilizing the elliptical machine during Pregnancy, listening to your body and avoiding overexerting yourself is vital. Start with a modest resistance and progressively raise it over time. It's also crucial to remain hydrated and take breaks as required.

Overall, the elliptical machine may be a safe and efficient option to keep active throughout your second trimester of

Pregnancy. As usual, it's vital to consult your healthcare professional before beginning any new fitness regimen.

3.2.2 Stationary bike

Stationary bikes are an excellent alternative for pregnant women who wish to be active throughout their second trimester. They give a low-impact cardiovascular exercise that is mild on the joints and can be readily changed to fit your changing demands.

One of the main benefits of utilizing a stationary bike is that it enables you to adjust the intensity of your exercise. You may modify the resistance and slope levels to enhance or reduce the intensity of your exercise, depending on how you feel that day. This makes it a perfect alternative for pregnant women who may suffer swings in energy levels and general Fitness during their Pregnancy.

In addition, stationary bikes are also a safe and pleasant alternative for pregnant women, as they offer a steady platform for exercise and support for the back and joints. This may be especially advantageous during the second trimester, as your baby and tummy continue to expand and move your center of gravity.

While utilizing a stationary bike throughout your second trimester, it is vital to make specific alterations to your training program. For example, you may need to elevate the handlebars to accommodate your developing belly and prevent leaning too far forward. It is also crucial to listen to your body and change the intensity of your exercise as required.

Overall, stationary bikes are an excellent alternative for pregnant women aiming to maintain their fitness levels throughout their second trimester. But be careful to contact your healthcare physician before beginning any new fitness regimen to verify it is safe for you and your baby.

3.3 Prenatal Yoga and Pilates for the second trimester

During the second trimester of Pregnancy, prenatal yoga and Pilates may be practical exercises for pregnant moms. Both workouts help strengthen and stretch the muscles, promote flexibility, and improve balance and posture. They may also help relieve stress and anxiety, which is vital for the mother's and baby's physical and emotional well-being.

Prenatal yoga and Pilates concentrate on Breathing methods and exercises suitable for pregnant women. These often contain moderate stretches, postures, and motions adapted to fit the changing body of the expecting woman. This implies that the exercises are meant to assist in easing typical pregnant discomforts such as back pain, swelling ankles, and tight muscles.

In prenatal yoga, pregnant moms learn to concentrate on their breath and connect with their bodies in a relaxing and meditative manner. The positions are generally practiced on a mat and may be changed to suit the mother's comfort level. Prenatal Pilates, on the other hand, focuses on strengthening core strength, which is vital for maintaining excellent posture and lowering the risk of back discomfort. The exercises in Pilates are typically done on a mat or a machine called a Reformer, which provides resistance to assist in developing the muscles.

It is crucial to know that not all yoga or Pilates courses are suited for pregnant women. Thus, searching for programs mainly created for prenatal yoga and Pilates is vital, or seeking instruction from a trained teacher with experience dealing with pregnant women is vital. With adequate instruction and adaptations, pregnant moms may safely practice prenatal yoga and Pilates to enhance their physical and mental health throughout the second trimester of Pregnancy.

Chapter Four:

4.0 Third Trimester Workout

4.1 Workout Adaptations for the third trimester

When you approach the third trimester of Pregnancy, changing your workout program to safeguard your and your baby's safety is crucial. Here are some workout adjustments to consider:

1. **Lower intensity:** Limit the intensity of your workouts and avoid high-impact activities. Instead, concentrate on low-impact workouts that put less stress on your joints.
2. **Shorter your workout:** Decrease the time of your exercises and take more regular breaks.
3. **Listen to your body:** Pay attention to how you feel throughout the exercises. If you experience any pain or discomfort, cease the workout and relax.
4. **Avoid laying on your back:** Avoid workouts that require you to rest on your back for a long time since this might limit blood supply to the uterus.

5. **Include extra stretching**: As your body changes, stretching is crucial to preserve flexibility and avoid muscular pain.
6. **Employ support**: Utilize props and support during workouts, such as a chair or stability ball, to maintain balance and prevent pressure on your back.
7. **Concentrate on Breathing:** Perform deep breathing techniques during exercise to assist in managing any pain and minimize tension.

Always speak with your healthcare physician before beginning or changing any fitness regimen during Pregnancy.

4.1.1 Reduce intensity

When exercising during the third trimester of Pregnancy, it's necessary to lower the intensity of your exercises. As your baby develops, your body is under increasing pressure, and you may suffer exhaustion, shortness of breath, and pain. High-impact sports like sprinting and leaping may no longer be comfortable or safe, so it's a good idea to transition to low-impact exercises that are gentler on your joints.

Even with low-impact activities, listening to your body and altering your training regimen as required is crucial. This may involve lowering your exercises' frequency, length, or intensity. Remember that it's normal to take breaks when needed and adapt routines as required to fit your changing physique.

Some recommended low-impact workouts to attempt during the third trimester are walking, swimming, and pregnancy yoga. These workouts help you maintain your Fitness and energy levels while lowering the chance of injury. Nonetheless, it's always a good idea to talk with your healthcare professional before beginning any new fitness regimen during Pregnancy, particularly in the latter stages.

4.1.2 Shorten your workout

Shortening your workout is a fantastic approach to adapting your fitness program during the third trimester of Pregnancy. As your baby develops, it might become tougher to maintain the same exercise level. By lowering the time of your exercises, you may still keep active without overexerting yourself.

While shortening your exercise, concentrate on quality above quantity. Instead of attempting to pack in as many exercises as possible, pick a few essential moves that target numerous muscle groups. This will help you get the most out of your exercise in a shorter period.

Try dividing your exercise into smaller, more doable parts throughout the day. For example, you may take a 10-minute exercise in the morning, another 10 minutes during your lunch break, and a final 10 minutes in the evening. This may help you keep consistent with your workout regimen while preventing weariness and pain.

Always listen to your body and alter your exercise as required. If you feel tired or uncomfortable, take a pause and relax. And remember to keep hydrated and feed your body with healthy meals to assist your baby's growth and development.

4.1.3 Listen to your body

Throughout the third trimester of Pregnancy, it's vital to listen to your body and alter your training regimen appropriately. Your body is going through substantial changes while your baby develops, and you may more readily suffer physical pain or exhaustion.

Pay attention to any indicators of discomfort or pain during exercise, and alter or stop the activity if required. This may involve lowering the intensity or length of your activity or moving to a lower-impact exercise.

Remember, the aim throughout this trimester is to maintain your fitness level and keep your body strong and healthy, not to push yourself to new boundaries or achieve personal records. Follow your instincts and prioritize your personal well-being and that of your developing kid.

4.1.4 Avoid sleeping on your back

As your pregnancy advances, avoiding reclining on your back during exercise is crucial. This is because the weight of your uterus and developing baby might strain the main blood arteries that carry oxygen and nourish your baby. This may lead to dizziness, lightheadedness, and a dip in blood pressure in rare circumstances.

Instead, choose workouts that enable you to remain upright or rest on your side. This includes activities like walking, swimming, and prenatal yoga. If you need to lie down, consider propping yourself up with pillows at a slight angle rather than flat on your back.

Always listen to your body and check with your healthcare practitioner before beginning any new fitness regimen during Pregnancy.

4.1.5 Include more stretching

As you go through your third trimester, you may notice that your body feels increasingly tight and unpleasant. Adding additional stretching to your training regimen may be a terrific method to release stress and lessen pain.

Moderate stretching exercises increase flexibility, decrease muscular tension, and enhance circulation. Moreover, stretching may help prepare your body for labor and Delivery by expanding your range of motion and improving your posture.

Some fantastic stretching exercises to integrate into your regimen during the third trimester are hip openers, pelvic tilts, and gentle twists. It's vital to remember to take things gently and not push yourself too hard since overstretching may be dangerous.

Always listen to your body and quit if you experience any discomfort or pain. Moreover, it's a good idea to consult your healthcare practitioner before starting any new workout plan, including stretching.

4.1.6 Use support

Throughout the third trimester of Pregnancy, the developing baby may place a lot of strain on your back and pelvic floor muscles. This may make activities more challenging and raise the risk of injury. To minimize this, it's suggested to employ assistance when exercising.

Support may come in numerous ways, such as utilizing a stability ball or a chair for balance during particular activities. You may also use a pregnancy support belt to relieve the strain off your back and improve posture. Support may help you be comfortable and safe while still obtaining excellent exercise during your third trimester.

It's vital to contact your healthcare physician before beginning any fitness regimen during Pregnancy and heed your body's demands.

4.1.7 Focus on Breathing

During the third trimester of Pregnancy, focusing on your breathing during exercise is essential. Proper breathing techniques can help you stay relaxed, calm, and focused during workouts. One way is to take slow, deep breaths through your nose and mouth. This may help you feel calmer and prevent you from becoming too winded during activity. It's also vital to avoid holding your breath when exercising, since this may raise your blood pressure and put additional strain on your heart.

4.2 Breathing Exercises for Labor and Delivery

Breathing exercises are a vital aspect of preparing for labor and Delivery. They may help manage pain and anxiety, decrease stress and tension, and improve relaxation. Different breathing methods expecting moms may utilize during labor and Delivery, including:

Deep Breathing entails taking slow, deep breaths through the nose and out through the mouth. It helps soothe the body and alleviate stress.

Slow Breathing: This method entails taking long, leisurely breaths in and out via the nose. It may assist in controlling pain and relieve anxiety.

Patterned Breathing: This method includes breathing for a specific number of counts, holding the breath for a given number, and expelling for a certain number of counts. It can help distract from the pain and increase relaxation.

Relaxation Breathing: This technique focuses on relaxing different body parts with each exhale. It can help manage pain and reduce tension.

Breathing exercises can be practiced throughout Pregnancy to become second nature by the time of labor and Delivery. They may also be utilized during other stressful moments, such as contractions during early labor or pushing during Delivery. It's crucial to consult with a healthcare physician or birthing instructor to understand and apply these strategies correctly.

4.2.1 Deep Breathing

Deep Breathing is a method that includes taking slow, deep breaths in through the nose and out through the mouth. It is commonly used in relaxation and meditation techniques to produce a feeling of calm and decrease tension and anxiety.

During labor and Delivery, deep Breathing may be an excellent technique to manage discomfort and remain focused. Ladies in labor may practice deep Breathing by taking slow, deep breaths in through their noses and then gently expelling them through their mouths. Some ladies find it beneficial to count to four as they inhale and six as they exhale to make their Breathing more regulated and regular.

Deep Breathing might also aid during the pushing stage of childbirth. Inhaling deeply and holding your breath for a few seconds before expelling might assist in building up pressure in the belly and make pushing more effective.

It is vital to highlight that deep breathing methods should be done throughout Pregnancy, not only during labor and Delivery, to grow familiar with the technique and to encourage relaxation and stress reduction. Talking with a healthcare expert before starting any new workout or breathing program during Pregnancy is vital.

4.2.2. Slow Breathing

Slow Breathing is a method that includes taking long, deep breaths and exhaling slowly. It may be a valuable tool for controlling tension, anxiety, and pain during labor and Delivery. To practice slow Breathing, select a comfortable posture, either sitting or lying down. Put one hand on your tummy and the other on your chest. Inhale gently through your nose, allowing your belly to expand and rise as you fill your lungs with air. Hold your breath for a few seconds, then exhale slowly through your mouth, allowing your tummy and chest to shrink as you release the air. Continue this pattern of slow Breathing for many minutes, concentrating on the sensations of the breath traveling in and out of your body. With practice, calm Breathing may become a valuable technique for relaxation and stress alleviation during labor and Delivery.

4.2.3 Patterned Breathing:

Patterned Breathing, also known as rhythmic Breathing, is a method that includes taking slow, deep breaths in a repeating sequence. This method is widely used during labor and Delivery to assist in controlling discomfort and enhance calm.

Various distinct types of patterned Breathing may be employed during childbirth. One popular pattern is the "slow breath," when the lady takes a big breath and then slowly exhales for a count of 5 or 6. Another pattern is "modified paced breathing," when the lady takes a big breath in and then exhales in a succession of little breaths, like blowing out candles.

Patterned Breathing may aid in relieving anxiety and stress during birth and diverting from pain. It may also aid in enhancing oxygen flow to the baby, which is crucial for fetal well-being.

It's crucial to practice patterned breathing methods before labor and Delivery to be utilized successfully throughout labor. Several childbirth education seminars give a teaching on patterned breathing methods, and women may also practice on their own at home.

4.2.4 Relaxation Breathing:

Relaxation breathing is a method used to alleviate tension and promote relaxation. This form of Breathing entails taking slow, deep breaths and exhaling slowly. During relaxation breathing, people often concentrate on their breath and relieve muscle tension.

In labor and Delivery, relaxation breathing may assist women in managing pain and decrease anxiety. By concentrating on their breath and utilizing relaxation methods, women may help their bodies relax and minimize the discomfort associated with contractions.

There are numerous sorts of relaxation breathing methods, including the following:

1. **Diaphragmatic Breathing:** This form includes deep inhaling and exhaling from the diaphragm. It is also known as belly breathing since it causes the belly to rise and fall with each breath.
2. **Progressive muscle relaxation:** This method includes tensing and relaxing various muscular

groups while concentrating on Breathing. This may assist in alleviating tension and encourage relaxation.

3. **Visualization:** This approach includes utilizing the power of imagination to envision a relaxing place or circumstance while concentrating on the breath.

Relaxation breathing may be learned and practiced before labor and Delivery to help women feel more prepared and secure. Engaging with a healthcare physician or qualified childbirth educator is crucial to guarantee optimal technique and safety throughout labor and Delivery.

4.3 Pelvic Floor Exercises for the third trimester

Pelvic floor exercises, often known as Kegel exercises, are helpful throughout Pregnancy, particularly in the third trimester. These exercises strengthen the pelvic floor muscles, which may weaken during Pregnancy and Delivery. Strengthening these muscles may help avoid incontinence and maintain the pelvic organs.

To conduct pelvic floor exercises:

1. Start by sitting or lying down in a comfortable posture.
2. Tighten your pelvic muscles as though you are attempting to halt the flow of pee.
3. Hold the contraction for a few seconds, then release and relax.
4. Continue this technique multiple times, aiming for 10-20 repetitions per session.

As you continue your Pregnancy, you may find it increasingly tough to conduct pelvic floor exercises while lying down. You may execute them while sitting or standing, utilizing a chair or countertop for support. It's vital to prevent overexerting oneself, so listen to your body and pause as required.

In addition to completing pelvic floor exercises, including other types of exercise in your third-trimester program is crucial. Low-impact exercises like walking, swimming, and prenatal yoga may help you maintain your Fitness and prepare your body for Delivery. Be essential to contact your healthcare practitioner before beginning any new workout plan.

Chapter Five

5.0 Low-Impact Workouts

5.1 Swimming and water aerobics for Pregnancy

Swimming and water aerobics are fantastic low-impact activities that are safe and helpful for pregnant women, especially during the third trimester. The buoyancy of the water helps decrease strain on the joints and may improve back discomfort, which is a typical complaint during Pregnancy.

Swimming also gives fantastic cardiovascular exercise, vital for maintaining excellent health for both mother and baby. Water aerobics courses, which feature a range of exercises conducted in the water, may also be a fun way to keep active and mingle with other pregnant women.

It is important to remember to take breaks as needed and not to overexert yourself in the water. Be essential to check with your healthcare professional before beginning any new fitness routine during Pregnancy.

5.2 Walking and Hiking during Pregnancy

Walking and hiking are excellent forms of exercise for pregnant women, particularly during the later stages of Pregnancy. They are low-impact activities that can help improve cardiovascular health, maintain muscle strength and tone, and promote healthy weight gain.

Walking is a simple and efficient technique to keep active throughout Pregnancy. It is straightforward to add to your routine. Depending on your fitness level and feelings, you may start with short walks and progressively increase your distance and intensity over time. Walking also helps to ease tension and anxiety, which may be particularly useful during Pregnancy.

Hiking is another fantastic choice for pregnant ladies who like being outside. It gives a more rigorous exercise compared to walking and may assist in improving balance and coordination. But, it's crucial to pick hiking paths that are acceptable for your fitness level and to prevent falls or accidents.

Walking and hiking help prepare your body for labor and Delivery by strengthening your legs and boosting your endurance. They also allow you to interact with nature and spend time outside before your little one comes. But, it's always crucial to speak to your healthcare practitioner before beginning any new fitness routine during Pregnancy to verify it is healthy for you and your baby.

Chapter Six:

6.0 High-Intensity Workouts

6.1 HIIT Exercises with Pregnancy

High-intensity interval training (HIIT) is a popular form of exercise that involves alternating short bursts of high-intensity exercise with periods of rest or low-intensity exercise. While HIIT can effectively improve cardiovascular Fitness and burn calories, it may not be the best option for pregnant women.

During Pregnancy, the body undergoes numerous changes that can affect a woman's ability to perform high-intensity exercise. These changes include an increase in blood volume, a decrease in lung capacity, and a shift in the body's center of gravity. Additionally, the hormones produced during Pregnancy can make joints and ligaments laxer, increasing the risk of injury.

For these reasons, pregnant women are generally not recommended to engage in a high-intensity exercise like HIIT. However, if a woman regularly participated in HIIT before becoming pregnant and has clearance from her healthcare provider, she may be able to continue with modifications.

These modifications may include decreasing the intensity and frequency of the workouts, increasing rest periods, and avoiding exercises that place to intensity of the exercise during Pregnancy. This may be done by lowering the weight lifted, the pace of the exercise, or the amount of resistance.

Avoid leaping or rapid movements: High-impact actions such as jumping or quick movements should be avoided during Pregnancy. This may raise the danger of harm or impair the baby's health.

Maintain the heart rate within a healthy range: Throughout Pregnancy, the heart rate should be kept within a safe range. A heart rate monitor may be used to ensure that the heart rate does not exceed the safe range.

Concentrate on low-impact activities: Low-impact exercises such as stationary cycling, swimming, or walking are safe alternatives to high-intensity workouts.

Please consult with a healthcare provider: It is vital to contact a healthcare professional before participating in high-intensity exercises during Pregnancy. They may recommend what adaptations to make and what workouts to avoid.

6.2.1 Decrease intensity

Lowering intensity is a necessary adaptation for high-intensity exercises during Pregnancy. Although high-intensity interval training (HIIT) may be a terrific approach to keeping active and maintaining Fitness throughout Pregnancy, it's crucial to make adaptations to protect the safety of both the mother and the baby.

Lowering intensity can be reduced by reducing the degree of resistance or weight used in exercises, shortening the session time, or decreasing the intensity of intervals. Allowing more excellent rest and recovery time between intervals and exercises is vital.

By lowering intensity, the exercise may still be challenging and effective without placing unnecessary pressure on the body. This change may also assist in minimizing overheating and tiredness, which can be problematic during Pregnancy.

It's crucial to listen to your body and talk with your healthcare physician to identify the proper intensity for your unique demands and fitness level during Pregnancy.

6.2.2. Avoid leaping or rapid movements

During Pregnancy, it's crucial to be careful when exercising, particularly with high-intensity exercises like HIIT (High-Intensity Interval Training) (High-Intensity Interval Training). One strategy to adapt these exercises is to avoid leaping or rapid movements that might stress your joints and raise the chance of damage. Instead, consider low-impact workouts, such as step-ups or lunges without leaps.

Another alteration to consider is to lessen the intensity of the exercise overall. Instead of pushing yourself to your limits, pause when required and lessen the weight or resistance utilized during workouts. This will still enable you to exercise solidly without putting extra stress on your body.

It's also crucial to pay attention to how your body is feeling throughout the exercise. Stop and take a break if anything doesn't seem right or you feel uncomfortable. Listen to your body and alter your exercise correctly to guarantee your and your baby's safety.

6.2.3 Maintain the heart rate within a safe range:

During Pregnancy, it's crucial to maintain your heart rate within a healthy range when exercising to prevent any possible complications. During high-intensity exercises, monitoring your heart rate and maintaining it below 140 beats per minute is advisable. Nevertheless, this figure may change based on your unique fitness level and pregnancy status, so it's essential to contact your healthcare professional for individualized assistance. Also, you may use a monitor to check your heart rate during exercise and alter your intensity appropriately to ensure you remain within a safe range.

6.2.4 Concentrate on low-impact exercises:

Throughout Pregnancy, it's crucial to concentrate on low-impact workouts to avoid the chance of injury or problems. This is particularly true for high-intensity activities when the risk of injury might be increased. Low-impact activities may assist in keeping you active and preserving cardiovascular health without placing too much stress on your body.

Some examples of low-impact exercises that may be integrated into high-intensity workouts with adjustments include:

Low-impact cardio: Instead of high-intensity jumping exercises, switch to low-impact cardio exercises such as walking, cycling, or using an elliptical machine.

Yoga or Pilates: These exercises can provide a low-impact workout that still helps to improve strength, flexibility, and balance. Make sure to choose classes designed explicitly for Pregnancy and avoid exercises requiring lying on your back or twisting.

Resistance band training: Resistance band training can effectively tone muscles and build strength without putting too much stress on your joints.

Swimming: Swimming is a low-impact workout that may assist in maintaining cardiovascular Fitness and muscular tone. It's also a great way to stay relaxed and comfortable during Pregnancy.

By incorporating these low-impact exercises into your high-intensity workout routine, you can still maintain Fitness and stay healthy during Pregnancy while reducing the risk of injury or complications. Always consult your healthcare provider before beginning any new exercise program during Pregnancy.

Chapter Seven:

7.0 Core Workouts for Pregnancy

7.1 The importance of core strength during Pregnancy

Maintaining core strength during Pregnancy is crucial for overall health and well-being. A strong core can help support the weight of the growing uterus, reduce back pain, and improve posture. It can also assist with labor and Delivery, making it easier to push during the second stage of labor.

However, it is essential to note that traditional core exercises like crunches and sit-ups may not be appropriate during Pregnancy. These exercises can put too much strain on the abdominal muscles and pelvic floor, which can weaken these areas and cause discomfort.

Instead, pregnant women can focus on gentle core exercises that engage the deep abdominal muscles and promote good posture. Some examples include pelvic tilts, cat-cow stretches, and modified planks.

Working with a certified prenatal fitness instructor or healthcare provider is also essential to ensure proper technique and safety during core exercises. Pregnant women should always listen to their bodies and modify exercises to avoid discomfort or pain.

7.2 Safe core exercises for each trimester

Maintaining core strength is essential during Pregnancy as it can help support the growing belly and prevent lower back pain. Unfortunately, not all core workouts are healthy for each trimester of Pregnancy. Here are some safe core exercises for each trimester:

First Trimester:

During the first trimester, it's vital to concentrate on easy core workouts that don't place too much pressure on the abdominal muscles. Safe workouts include:

Pelvic tilts: Lay on your back with your legs bent and feet flat on the ground. Gently tilt your pelvis up and down while working your core muscles.

Modified plank: Get into a plank posture with your knees on the ground instead of your toes. Maintain this posture for a few seconds while working your core muscles.

Second Trimester:

During the second trimester, avoiding workouts that entail laying on your back is crucial. Safe workouts include:

Cat-cow stretch: Go on your hands and knees and alternate between arching your back up like a cat and rounding it down like a cow.

Standing core twists: Stand with your feet hip-width apart and twist your upper body side to side while using your core muscles.

Third Trimester:

During the third trimester, avoiding exercises that put too much strain on the abdominal muscles is essential. Safe workouts include:

Sitting marches: Sit on a stability ball or chair and alternate raising each leg while activating your core muscles.

Kegels: Kegel exercises include tightening and releasing the pelvic floor muscles. These activities assist in preparing for labor and Delivery.

It's crucial to listen to your body throughout each trimester and adapt routines as required. If you encounter any pain or discomfort, cease the activity immediately and talk with your healthcare physician.

Chapter Eight

8.0 Prenatal Yoga

8.1 Benefits of prenatal yoga

Prenatal yoga is a mild kind of exercise that is mainly developed for pregnant women. It contains a sequence of postures, breathing exercises, and meditation methods that may enable women to remain healthy, flexible, and comfortable throughout their Pregnancy.

There are several advantages of prenatal yoga, including:

Decreased stress: Pregnancy may be difficult, but prenatal yoga can assist women in relaxing and lowering their stress levels.

Increased flexibility: Prenatal yoga may enable women to retain flexibility throughout Pregnancy, which can help prepare the body for labor and Delivery.

Decreased back pain: Many pregnant women feel back pain. However, prenatal yoga may assist to relieve this discomfort.

Increased circulation: Prenatal yoga may assist in enhancing circulation, which can benefit the health of both the mother and the baby.

Decreased risk of difficulties: Frequent prenatal yoga practice has been associated with a reduced risk of specific issues during Pregnancy, including high blood pressure and gestational diabetes.

Better sleep: Pregnancy may make obtaining a good night's sleep difficult, but prenatal yoga can assist women in relaxing and sleeping better.

Better posture: As the baby develops, many pregnant women have poor posture, but prenatal yoga may assist in improving posture and avoiding pain.

Connecting with the baby: Prenatal yoga may be a terrific method for women to connect with their unborn babies and prepare for the bonding experience of parenthood.

Overall, prenatal yoga may be a safe and effective approach for pregnant women to keep both physically and psychologically well. It is vital to check with a healthcare physician before starting any fitness program during Pregnancy and to work with a competent prenatal yoga teacher who can lead you through safe and suitable postures and adjustments for each trimester.

8.2 Prenatal yoga postures for each trimester

Prenatal yoga is a terrific method for pregnant women to keep active, decrease stress, and prepare their bodies for birth and Delivery. Yoga may also help ease typical pregnant symptoms such as back discomfort, exhaustion, and sleeplessness. Yet, it's vital to alter positions during each trimester to suit your expanding belly and changing physique.

First Trimester:

Throughout the first trimester, it's vital to concentrate on moderate postures that support your developing body without placing too much pressure on your muscles. Some friendly stances to attempt include:

Cat-cow stance: This pose helps to gently extend the spine and reduce stress in the lower back.

Modified pigeon position: This stance helps open the hips and stretch the glutes.

Sitting forward fold: This position helps to stretch the hamstrings and lower back while boosting circulation.

Warrior II stance: This pose helps to increase strength in the legs and core while opening up the hips.

Second Trimester:

During the second trimester, avoiding positions that entail laying on your back or belly is recommended. It's also vital to avoid positions that exert too much strain on the abdominal muscles. Some friendly stances to attempt include:

Triangle position: This stance helps open the hips and stretch the hamstrings.

Tree pose: This pose helps to improve balance and strengthen the legs.

Half pigeon stance: This pose helps to extend the hips and reduce tension in the lower back.

Cobra posture: This stance helps strengthen the back and open the chest.

Third Trimester:

Throughout the third trimester, avoiding positions that entail deep twisting or backbends is crucial. Avoiding positions that place too much strain on the pelvic floor is vital. Some friendly stances to attempt include:

Modified goddess position: This posture helps open the hips and strengthen the legs.

Side-lying savasana: This position helps release back stress and promote circulation.

Bound angle position: This pose helps to extend the hips and reduce tension in the lower back.

Sitting cat-cow stance: This pose helps to gently extend the spine and reduce tension in the lower back.

Overall, prenatal yoga may give several advantages throughout Pregnancy, including stress reduction, greater flexibility and strength, and preparation for labor and Delivery. But, it's vital to contact your healthcare professional before beginning any new fitness program and to alter positions as required during each trimester.

8.3 Adjustments for typical pregnancy problems

Throughout Pregnancy, women may suffer several physical changes and concerns. It is vital to alter activities to suit these changes and prevent increasing any pain or difficulties. These are some frequent pregnancy issues and adaptations for exercise:

Round ligament pain: This is a frequent ache during Pregnancy owing to the stretching of the ligaments that support the uterus. To prevent increasing this discomfort, avoid rapid movements and opt for low-impact workouts like walking, swimming, and prenatal yoga.

Back discomfort: As the baby develops, it may strain the lower back, producing pain. Avoid workouts requiring leaping or rapid movements, and concentrate on low-impact activities that strengthen the back muscles, such as swimming and prenatal Pilates.

Pelvic discomfort: Some women may suffer pain in the pelvic region during Pregnancy due to hormonal changes that loosen the ligaments and joints in the area. Avoid workouts requiring broad leg motions or deep squats, and choose exercises that strengthen the pelvic floor muscles, such as Kegels.

High blood pressure or gestational diabetes: These disorders need constant monitoring by a healthcare professional, and it may be required to appropriately change the intensity and kind of exercise. Collaborate with a healthcare physician or licensed prenatal fitness instructor to design a safe and effective workout regimen.

Fatigue: Many women suffer exhaustion throughout Pregnancy, especially in the first and third trimesters. It is crucial to listen to your body and relax when required. Reduce workouts by lowering intensity, lessening the activity time, or choosing low-impact activities like walking or pregnancy yoga.

Always speak with a healthcare physician before beginning any fitness program during Pregnancy and make changes as required to ensure a safe and pleasant workout.

Chapter Nine

9.0 Diet and Exercise

9.1 Nutritional demands during pregnancy

Nutrition is vitally crucial during Pregnancy to promote the growth and development of the child, as well as the health and well-being of the mother. These are some essential dietary demands and issues during Pregnancy:

Protein: Protein is needed for the growth and development of the fetus, as well as the production of breast milk following Delivery. Pregnant women should strive to take 70-100 grams of protein daily from lean meats, poultry, fish, eggs, dairy products, beans, and nuts.

Folate: Folate is necessary for forming the neural tube, forming the baby's brain and spinal cord. Pregnant women should strive to eat 600-800 mcg of folate daily from foods such as leafy green vegetables, citrus fruits, beans, and fortified cereals.

Iron: Iron is needed to develop red blood cells supplying oxygen to the infant. Pregnant women should strive to ingest

27 mg of iron daily from lean meats, chicken, fish, beans, and fortified cereals.

Calcium: Calcium is vital for developing the baby's bones and teeth and helps preserve the mother's bone health. Pregnant women should strive to eat 1000-1300 mg of calcium daily from dairy products, leafy green vegetables, fortified soy products, and calcium-fortified beverages.

Omega-3 fatty acids: Omega-3 fatty acids are vital for developing the baby's brain and vision. Pregnant women should strive to ingest 200-300 mg of omega-3 fatty acids daily from sources such as fatty fish (like salmon), flaxseed, chia seeds, and walnuts.

Hydration: Pregnant women must keep well-hydrated to promote the health and development of the baby, as well as to help avoid constipation and urinary tract infections. Pregnant women should strive to take at least 8-10 cups of water each day and may require more if they are active or in hot weather.

Avoid specific foods: Pregnant women should avoid foods detrimental to the growing baby, including raw or undercooked meat, poultry, or fish; unpasteurized dairy products; and raw or undercooked eggs. They should also reduce their consumption of caffeine and avoid alcohol and smoking.

Pregnant women must engage with their healthcare professional to ensure they achieve their particular dietary demands throughout Pregnancy. Some women may also benefit from prenatal vitamins to help fill nutritional shortfalls.

9.2 How to fuel your exercises when pregnant

Throughout Pregnancy, it's crucial to nourish your body appropriately for your and your developing baby's health. When it comes to exercise, an appropriate diet may give you the energy and nutrients your body needs to perform efficiently and recuperate correctly. Here are some recommendations on how to feed your activities while pregnant:

Keep hydrated: Consuming adequate water is vital for general health and optimal body functioning during activity. Drink 8-10 glasses of water daily, and even more if you exercise. Try taking a water bottle with you to sip on throughout the day.

Eat a balanced diet: Be sure to consume various nutrient-dense meals to give your body the energy and resources it needs to function correctly throughout exercises. This contains lean protein, complex carbs, healthy fats, and various fruits and vegetables.

Timing your meals and snacks: Eating before and after exercises may assist in supplying the required energy and nutrients for your body. Try to have a small meal or snack containing carbs and protein 30 minutes to an hour before exercising and another small meal or snack within 30 minutes to an hour after exercising.

Listen to your body: Heed your hunger signals and ate when hungry. It's also crucial to relax when you need it and avoid overexerting yourself.

Consider talking with a licensed dietitian: A certified dietitian can help you establish a tailored nutrition plan that suits your particular requirements and supports your fitness program throughout Pregnancy.

Remember, it's vital to consult your healthcare practitioner before beginning or modifying your workout regimen and eating plan during Pregnancy.

First Trimester Workout Plan

Week1	01 **Leg supersets** 25minutes	02 **Arm+Abs Supersets** 25Minutes	03 **Low impact HIIT** 30Minutes	04 **Prenatal Abs or barre** class 10-20Minutes	05 **Full body kettlebell** 30Minutes
Week2	06 **Legs+Butt** 40Minutes	07 **Arm+Back** 25Minutes	08 **Legs+Shoulder** 35Minutes	**09** **Hip Flexor Stretch and Beginners Abs** 15Minutes	10 **Kettlebell Legs** 30Minutes
Week3	11 **Leg Supersets** 20Minutes	12 **Arm+Abs Supersets** 25Minutes	13 **Low Impact HIIT** 20Minutes	14 **Cardio+Unliteral Strength** 40Minutes	15 **Full Body Strength** 30Minutes
Week4	16 **Legs+Butt** 40Minutes	17 **Chest+Arm** 25Minutes	18 **Leg and Walk Or Jog and Mobility** 10minutes	19 **Full Body Strength Training** 35Minutes	20 **Beginner Abs** 15Minutes

Second Trimester Workout Plan

	01	02	03	04	05
W k 1	**Leg Superset s** 30Minute s	**Back+Bice ps** 25Minutes	**Full Body Strength+Card io** 35Miutes	**Low imoack Strength + Cardio** 20Minute s	**Low Impack Cardio Barre** 15 Minutes
	06	07	08	09	10
W k 2	**Lower Body** 30Minute s	**Chest, Shoulder Biceps** 25Minutes	**Prenatal Arms+Prenatal Legs** 25Minutes	**Prenatal Barre** 25Minute s	**Standing Abs** 10- 20Minute s
	11	12	13	14	15
W k 3	**Legs Superset s** 30Minute s	**Full Body Strength+ Cardio** 35Minutes	**Low Impact Strength+ Cardio** 20Minutes	**Prenatal Abs or back Stretch** 10- 20Minute s	**Low Impact cardio Barre** 15Minute s
	16	17	18	19	20
W k 4	**Lower Body** 30Minute s	**Chest Shoulder+ Triceps** 20Minutes	**Prenatal Barre** 25Minutes	**Body Weight Prenatal** 35Minute s	**Prenatal Arm and Prenatal Legs** 25Minute s

Third Trimester Workout Plan

Wk1	01	02	03	04	05
	Full Body Strength 30Minutes	**Prenatal Legs and Prenatal Cardio** 35Minutes	**Dumbbell Arm** 30Minutes	**Pregnancy Barre** 20Minutes	**Rest Day**
Wk2	06	07	08	09	10
	Prenatal Pilates And Back Stretch 20Minutes	**Advance pregnancy Workout** 30Minutes	**Prenatal Yoga Flow** 15Minutes	**Rest Day**	**Rest Day**
Wk3	11	13	14	15	16
	Prenatal Legs and Prenatal Cardio 25minutes	**SPD Stretch** 15Minutes	**Rest Day**	**Rest Day**	**Rest Day**
Wk4	17	18	19	20	21
	Prenatal Yoga 25Minutes	**Advanced Pregnancy Workout** 30minutes	**Prenatal Pilates + Cardio** 35minutes	**Rest Day**	**Rest Day**